An Inn

MW00441718

Technology

15 Simple Steps to Dropping Pounds in a Matter of Days.

Based on the science of how the body needs to be fed and exercised in order to function optimally while losing weight, this Itty Bitty Book is filled with vital information. It uses the body's own chemistry to lose pounds.

Examples:

- Eating one bite of protein first at every meal.
- Limiting your carbohydrate intake to below 60 grams per day.
- Counting Carbs not Calories!

If reading big diet books is not your thing, grab a copy of this little book, just follow the chapter headings and start losing weight today.

Reviews

Love this book! Helpful hints for busy people
written by a leading expert in health and fitness.
Clear and concise, it gives you step by step
helpful tips for staying on track and making your
health a top priority. I would highly recommend
this wonderful itty bitty book!

By Rosemary Gullizia Workman

Your Amazing
Itty Bitty®

Weight Loss Book

15 Simple Steps to Weight Loss Success

Suzy Prudden
And
Joan Meijer-Hirschland

Published by Itty Bitty® Publishing
A subsidiary of S & P Productions, Inc.

Printed in the United States of America

Itty Bitty® Publishing
311 Main Street, Suite D
El Segundo, CA 90245
(310) 640-8885

ISBN: 978-1-931191-05-0

Dedicated to our children

Rob Sussman, Peter Meijer, Richard Meijer, Jacqueline Kreple.

Stop by our Itty Bitty® website to find interesting blog entries regarding How to Lose Weight Easily and Effortlessly.

www.IttyBittyPublishing.com

Table of Contents

90g. carb/day for brain /glucose
blood sugar

The Simple Steps

Step 1
Eat a Maximum of 60-Grams of
Carbohydrates Daily

You can eat all the fresh green vegetables you
want as long as you stay under 60 grams and
above 45 grams of carbohydrates each day.

1. Select from complex carbohydrates.
2. Avoid starches (simple carbohydrates).
   Starches metabolize as sugar and store as
   fat.
3. Starches also trigger insulin release so
   your body can't burn fat for four hours
   after you eat them.
4. Starches aren't necessary for healthy
   living. Complex carbohydrates (aka
   green vegetables) are necessary.
5. Green vegetables supply vitamins,
   minerals, enzymes and fiber.
6. The rule of thumb with carbohydrates is:
   "Eat nothing white, except cauliflower,
   garlic and members of the mushroom and
   onion families."

Include: Complex Carbohydrates:

- Asparagus ½ cup: 1 gram carbohydrate.
- Broccoli (½ cup): 6 grams carbohydrate.
- Cauliflower (½ cup): 5 grams carbohydrate.
- Peppers (½ cup): 6.5 grams carbohydrate.
- Onions (½ cup): 1 gram carbohydrate.
- Green beans (½ cup): 4 grams carbohydrate.

Avoid: Simple Carbohydrates (aka Starches):

Pepp. Farm Original 13g. Carb

- Bread (slice): 34 grams carbohydrate.
- Bagel (1 whole white): 59 grams carbohydrate.
- French fries (small serving): 32.7 grams carbohydrate.
- Pizza (small slice): 20 grams carbohydrate.
- Baked potato (plain): 29.6 grams carbohydrate.

Dave's Thin Slice Good Seed Brd
13g. carb/slice
Steel cut oatmeal from Oberweis
30g. carb/serving
Cheerios plain, 2 0.75c., 15g.
Oatmeal old-fashioned, ½c., 28g.

Step 2
Avoid Empty Carbohydrates

Processed foods are regarded as empty carbohydrates, they contribute to your carbohydrate intake, but they do not contribute fiber, vitamins, minerals or the enzymes your body requires for optimum health.

1. Avoid all processed foods – like white flour, white pasta, white rice and all forms of sugar (including brown and "natural" sugars, honey and maple syrup).
2. If food comes in a box or a can avoid it.
3. The more food is processed, the fewer nutrients it contains. In varying degrees, all processed foods metabolize as sugar and store as fat.
4. Storage and travel also kills these important nutrients.
5. It is better to eat fresh, fiber-rich, vitamin- and mineral-packed green or colored vegetables for your carbohydrate choices.
6. Eat the colored vegetables fresh, raw, baked, broiled or lightly steamed if possible.
7. Avoid boiling and frying.

Include:

- Fresh, alive vegetables.
- Locally grown foods.
- Preferably from the farmers market or your garden.
- Cereals, like original oatmeal, that take 20 minutes or more to cook.

Avoid:

- All processed packaged, canned and frozen foods.
- Cake, cookie and bread mixes of all kinds.
- Cakes, cookies, pies, candy, white potatoes, white rice, grits, all boxed cereals, breads of all kinds, rolls, all pastas, tortillas (wheat, corn, rice, etc.), white flour (indeed all wheat products), corn bread and flour – all corn products.
- All foods containing MSG including products that say "Natural Flavors." MSG hides the poor quality of the foods it accompanies.
- Avoid all sugars, corn syrup, molasses, and artificial-sweeteners of all kind.
- Avoid any ingredients you can't pronounce.
- Avoid "Energy" Bars.

2oz meal = 14 g. protein x6 = 42g.

Step 3
Eat 28 Grams of Protein *= 84g./day*
Three Times Daily

Your body needs a constant supply of protein during the day.

1. Eat 28 grams of protein at each meal, three times a day.
2. Eat protein three times a day so your body doesn't steal protein from your lean muscle mass.
3. Losing lean muscle mass makes it harder to burn fat.
4. 28-grams equal the size of pack of playing cards, the palm of your hand or 3 eggs. *21 g, = 3 Eggs*
5. AVOID proteins combined with carbohydrates - buns and sauces. They are empty carbohydrates.
6. Eat breakfast and eat protein for breakfast. To lose weight keep protein levels constant throughout the day!
7. Skipping meals – and starvation diets – lowers your metabolism, which is counter-productive in weight loss.
8. Starvation diets cause you to lose water and muscle mass. It lowers your metabolism. Eat right to lose weight!

Include:

- Chicken, roasted or poached 0 grams carbohydrates.
- Turkey, roasted 0 grams carbohydrates.
- Lamb, 0 grams carbohydrates.
- Wild Salmon, 0 grams carbohydrates.
- Beef & Veal, 0 grams carbohydrates.

Avoid:

- Quarter Pounder with Cheese, 41 grams carbohydrates.
- Hot dog, on bun 23 grams carbohydrates.
- McDonald's Bacon Clubhouse, Crispy Chicken, 65 grams carbohydrates.
- All Meat Pizza, one slice, 30 grams carbohydrates.

A good rule is *"Eat One Bite of Protein Before Eating Anything Else At Each Meal."* Eating protein first sends a message to your body notifying your cells that their needs are being recognized and met.

Step 4
Eat Healthy Oils

Omega 3 and 6 Oils are essential for your health. They are called essential fatty acids.

1. At every meal eat one tablespoon of healthy oil (Omega 3 and Omega 6 oils in particular).
2. People on low fat diets have been known to lose so much energy they have become bedridden.
3. Avoid all products that say "hydrogenated" and "partially hydrogenated" on the labels.
4. Hydrogenated oils are fats that have been processed with extreme heat and toxic chemicals equivalent to Drano.
5. The safest oils are virgin olive oil, cold pressed flaxseed or other healthy cold pressed oils. Avoid any supermarket oils.
6. Avoid all margarines and shortenings which have been bombarded with heavy metals as well as heat and chemicals.
7. Omega 3 oil (from fish or flaxseed) is vital for heart and brain health.
8. Farm-fed fish do not supply healthy oils.
9. Limit your fats to 3 tablespoons a day.

Include:

- Oils in dark glass, black plastic or metal containers only.
- Olive oil, Flaxseed oil, fish oil, oil combinations of Omega 3, 6 and 9 essential fatty acids and butter are good oils to eat, but not to cook with.
- Cold pressed oils.
- Palm Oil handles heat the best of all oils.
- Never cook with Omega 3 oil (i.e. flaxseed or fish oil) which is extremely fragile. Use Coconut or Palm oil.
- Take your daily oil in liquid form rather than capsules (i.e. as in home made salad dressing).
- It takes 16 capsules to equal one tablespoon of oil. That's a lot of unnecessary gelatin.
- Keep your oils refrigerated after opening.

Avoid:

- All Supermarket oils – in clear glass or plastic containers.
- All hydrogenated or partially hydrogenated oils, margarines and shortenings.
- All cake, pie, pancake, muffin, bread and other mixes that contain hydrogenated oils.
- In particular avoid all low fat diets and products which contain lots of sugar.

Step 5
Eat Fiber Every Day

You've heard about fiber – it's what doesn't digest from the food you eat.

1. Fiber lowers cholesterol and keeps your intestines clean; it's an absolute MUST for your diet.
2. Lettuce (excluding iceberg, which is mostly water), carrots, celery and most green or colored vegetables are filled with fiber.
3. The quickest way to get lots of fiber, plus Omega 3 oil, is to eat three tablespoons of freshly ground flaxseed every day.
4. Whole flaxseed does not digest well so use only ground flaxseed.
5. You can add flaxseed to smoothies; sprinkle it on cottage cheese, cereals, vegetables, even eggs.
6. Use your coffee grinder to grind it freshly every day or the oil will spoil.
7. Do not use pre-ground flaxseed if you can avoid it. If you can't avoid it keep it refrigerated.

Include (but do not limit yourself to):

- Asparagus.
- Cabbage.
- Carrots.
- Cauliflower.
- Celery.
- Collard Greens.
- Beans.
- Beets plus Beet or Turnip Greens.
- Brussels Sprouts.
- Egg Plant.
- Flaxseed.
- Kale.
- Lettuce, all kinds.
- Mustard Greens (hot).
- Parsnips.
- Peppers.
- Radishes.
- Spinach.
- Sprouts of all kinds.
- Squashes, all kinds.
- String beans.
- Sweet Peas.
- Sweet Potatoes.

Avoid

- White Potatoes.
- White rice.
- Corn and corn products.
- Grains and grain products.

10

Step 6
Eat Organic

Non-organic produce is laced with pesticides, herbicides and fungicides that stores in your body fat. The more toxic the food you eat the more fat you need for storage.

1. Eat organic whenever possible.
2. Simply by shifting to organic, you can lose 20 pounds of protective fat in a year.
3. Inorganic meat is filled with growth hormones.
4. The hormones in meat and milk are causing our children to start puberty below the age of ten.
5. Inorganic meats and milk are also filled with antibiotics, which is destroying the effectiveness of life-saving antibiotics.
6. Don't let money sabotage your weight loss plan. If you feel you can't afford organic, stay with supermarket products or better yet grow your own garden.
7. If you can – buy locally at farmer's markets and eat foods in season when possible.
8. Farmer's markets not only support your health, but they support healthy land-use as well. Land that produces income is less likely to be sold for development.

Include:

- Organic vegetables.
- Grass fed beef and lamb.
- Free range poultry.
- Fish caught in the wild (not farm-raised).
- Organic fruit.

Note: Check label information because Big Agra is known to mislabel – calling non-organic foods organic by using loopholes provided by the FDA.

Avoid:

- Non-organic fruits, vegetables and meats.
- Non-organic Peaches treated with pesticides.
- Apples – which are coated with wax for that shiny glow.
- Farmed fish.
- Fish and shrimp grown in Asia.
- All foods grown outside of the USA.
- "Fresh" produce treated with chemicals to give them shelf life.
- Food which has been microwaved and GMOs – (genetically modified) like all soy products and zucchini.
- All food grown in China.
- Fruits and vegetables flown in from other countries where they are in-season. Travel kills vitamins and enzymes.

Step 7
Eat Fresh Foods

Eat foods that are fresh and cooked as little as possible (except meats which should be baked, broiled or boiled thoroughly).

1. Eat nothing fried.
2. Fresh and raw vegetables contribute vitamins, minerals and enzymes to your body.
3. Be sure to wash all fruits and vegetables thoroughly before you eat them.
4. Cold pressed oils feed your cells and enhance your metabolism. Heating destroys these vital nutrients.
5. Microwaving kills vitamins and enzymes.
6. Rule of thumb: If a process kills germs, it also kills vitamins and enzymes.

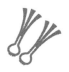

Include:

- Nuts (no more than 6-8 between meals).
- Salads (with healthy oil and vinegar dressing).
- Sprouts of all kinds.
- Steamed vegetables.
- Stewed meats.
- Roasted meats.
- Baked meats.
- Baked fish.
- Steamed fish.
- Baked, stewed or roasted poultry.

Avoid:

- Boiling.
- Frying.
- Commercial dressings.
- Fruits and Vegetables out of season.

Step 8
Read Labels

Labels will tell you how many sugars and how many carbohy-drates there are, in a package. They are designed to be confusing, but they will tell you at least that.

1. Don't eat things you can't pronounce.
2. Eat nothing processed. Processed foods contain heavy doses of sugar or salt, or both, neither of which is good for you.
3. Processing is the breaking down of food so that it most closely resembles a simple carbohydrate – exactly what you want to avoid.
4. Processed foods metabolize as sugar, which stores as fat.
5. Processed foods now contain high fructose corn syrup, which is much worse for your body than all other sugars.
6. Remember this mantra – simple carbohydrates metabolize as simple sugars. Processed foods turn into sugar and store as fat.
7. Avoid anything that is labeled "Low Fat." Low fat = high sugar.
8. "Natural Flavor," = MSG which tricks your mind into thinking healthy & fresh.
9. MSG is known to create serious allergies.

Include:

- Fresh foods that don't require labels.

Avoid:

- All items on a label you can't pronounce.
- High Fructose Corn Syrup.
- Hydrogenated and partially hydrogenated oils.
- Products in which the first item is sugar in any of its many names – dextrose, fructose, etc.
- MSG.
- Natural Flavors.
- All "Low Fat" products.

Step 9
Drink Water

Drink at least eight 8-ounce glasses of water a day.

1. Avoid soda, coffee, black tea, fruit juices and milk. Stick to water.
2. Nothing else is water.
3. Water does all kinds of good things for your body. You can lose up to 23 pounds in one year simply by switching from soda (diet or regular) to water.
4. Depending on how much fat it contains, your body is more than half water. It needs water to replace the water that is excreted through sweat and other means.
5. Water helps your body remove fat.
6. It protects you against osteoporosis.
7. It has zero carbs and zero calories.
8. For extra benefit, add a little fresh lemon or lime juice. (Don't use fake lemon or lime juice.)
9. Drinks that contain caffeine actually act as diuretics.
10. To offset the effects of one can of soda, you need to drink 2500 glasses of water.
11. Soda robs calcium from the bones – thus contributing to osteoporosis.

Include:

- Fresh water with fresh lemon (not fake lemon juice) added.

Avoid:

- All drinks that are not water.
- Soda uses vast amounts of water to create a toxic drink that not only harms your body but fails to hydrate it.
- Coffee is actually a diuretic.
- Water in plastic bottles.

Note: Plastic bottles contain a cancer causing BPA – Make absolutely certain you do not freeze water in plastic bottles or drink water that has been left in hot cars.

Step 10
Avoids

Avoid fruit juices, sports drinks, energy drinks, and soft drinks, even those that are low-cal or no-cal.

1. The problem is not only about calories, it's about chemicals and the way the body is stimulated to release insulin even when you are not using sugar directly.
2. Diet drinks may not have carbohydrates but they are just as bad as non-diet drinks.
3. Diet drinks cause fat to adhere to your cells.
4. They stimulate the pancreas to release insulin. Once insulin is circulating in your bloodstream, _you cannot physically burn fat for the next four hours_.
5. If aspartame gets heated, it turns into formaldehyde. Diet drinks are stored in un-air conditioned warehouses and carried in un-air conditioned trucks.
6. Equal is known to cause brain tumors.
7. Splenda, chemically tortured sugar, causes enlarged liver and kidneys.
8. Stevia is a good choice. It is an unaltered sweet leaf from the Andes Mountains.

Include:

- Water.
- Herbal tea.
- Hot lemon water.
- Stevia.

Avoid:

- Artificial sweetener.
- Diet Drinks of all kinds.
- Soft drinks with sugar.
- Fruit Juices.
- Coffee.
- Black Teas.
- Sports Drinks.
- Vitamin Drinks.

Step 11
How to Drink Coffee

If you must drink coffee (or black tea), drink it right after or with a protein-rich, fresh green vegetable and healthy-fat meal or snack.

1. Taken without a meal, coffee is recognized as a meal on its own.
2. Coffee consumed without food stimulates your adrenal glands for a fight-or-flight reaction.
3. Fight-or-flight stimulates your liver to release stored sugar for instant energy.
4. This, in turn, stimulates your pancreas to release insulin.
5. This means you can't burn fat for four hours after drinking a single cup of coffee.
6. The processing that results in De-Caf coffee makes this drink more harmful than caffeinated coffee.
7. In addition, coffee is a very oily bean.
8. Oil retains pesticides, herbicides and fungicides. Drink organic coffee when possible.

Include:

- Water.
- Water with Lemon.

Avoid:

- Non-organic coffees and teas.
- De-Caffeinated coffees and teas.
- Hot Chocolate.
- Black Tea.

Step 12
The Benefits of Exercise

Exercise for 5-20 minutes every morning.

1. Exercising in the morning sets your metabolism higher for the entire day.
2. Exercise can be as simple as walking up and down the driveway; but walk – don't stroll.
3. Walking is an aerobic exercise. It is great for heart health. It is not as good as weighted exercise for weight loss.
4. The most important thing to know about exercise is to start where you are.
5. If you have not exercised in years you cannot run the Decathlon the first day.
6. Our rule is that there is no gain in pain. As soon as your body starts to hurt, stop what you are doing and exercise another part of the body. There is no gain in pain.
7. Exercising to music that you really like is the best way to work out. Music makes you want to move, it requires that you keep time to a rhythm, it enforces pace.
8. Use positive suggestions as you exercise to keep your mind focused on improving instead of reinforcing complaints.

"I'm getting better and stronger every day in every way."

Include:

- Exercise.
- Exercise is the single most effective tool for reversing Diabetes and Heart Disease.
- If you do nothing else, exercise.

Avoid:

- Sitting without a break (as bad as smoking).

Step 13
Weighted Exercise and Lean Muscle Mass

Three times a week add weighted exercise to your regimen.

1. Weighted exercise builds lean muscle mass.
2. Muscle mass burns fat – even while you sleep.
3. You don't need fancy weights. A heavy book or unopened soup cans will do the trick.
4. Adding weights to your ankles and wrists while you walk can be highly effective as well. Keep the weights light, 1 to 2 pounds only.
5. Weighted exercises have the added benefit of preventing osteoporosis.
6. Bones respond to weight by increasing strength and density.
7. Weighted exercise is not aerobics. Aerobics is exercise for your heart muscle. It does not build fat burning muscle mass.

Include

- Weighted Exercise to your daily routine to build Lean Muscle mass.
- Lean Muscle burns fat.

Step 14
Take Vitamin and Enzyme Supplements

Because of the way our foods are grown and processed, the food you buy today has less than half the nutrition of the foods grown in 1950.

1. Time, travel and processing destroy vitamins and enzymes.
2. Your body functions are dependent on vitamins, minerals and enzymes.
3. Simply put, you need supplements.
4. Because you will be releasing toxins from your fat as you lose weight, it is important to take antioxidant vitamins and minerals every day.
5. Antioxidants attach to the toxins and help remove them from your system before they can attach to your cells and do damage.
6. Take a multivitamin-mineral combo.
7. Add a digestive enzyme supplement to your daily diet.
8. Cooking and processing destroys vitamins and enzymes without which certain bodily functions cannot take place.
9. Storage and transportation depletes vitamins and enzymes.

Include:

- Supplements Daily.
  - Vitamin.
  - Mineral.
  - Antioxidants.
  - Essential Fatty Acid.
  - Digestive Enzymes.
- Shopping at farmer's markets, and eating fresh foods in season, supports local farmers and supports your health.
- It impacts on land use all at the same time. Land that is profitable is less likely to be sold for development.
- If you grow your own hydroponic garden minerals and vitamins are included in the growth solution.

Step 15
Take Mineral Supplements

If you look at what minerals do in your body you would stop saying "vitamins and minerals," and say, "minerals and vitamins."

1. Big Agra replaces only three of the minerals that are stripped from the soil every year simply by the process of growing food.
2. It does not replace important trace minerals like zinc which are almost completely absent from American soil and therefore the American diet.
3. Minerals are absolutely vital to your health and well-being.
4. Fossil fuel fertilizers prevent soil from breaking down and releasing minerals into the soil.
5. If the minerals aren't in the soil, they don't get into the plants and they are no longer delivered to you through your diet.
6. Small amounts of trace minerals are vitally important.
7. Two important minerals that are sadly lacking from our soil are zinc and chromium which may be linked to the development of Type II Diabetes.

Include:

- A full spectrum supplement of minerals daily. Which include:
  - Calcium.
  - Magnesium.
  - Potassium.
  - Trace minerals.
  - Zinc.

Note: the Recommended Daily Amount of vitamins and minerals refers to the absolute minimum you require to prevent serious disease. It is a minimal, not an optimal, measurement.

You've finished. Before you go…

Tweet/share that you finished this book.
Please star rate this book.
Reviews are solid gold to writers. Please
take a few minutes to give us some itty
bitty feedback on this book.

About The Authors

SUZY PRUDDEN made her stage debut in a dance recital at the age of two as the lead elephant in a long line of two-year olds in a rendition of "The Circus." It was love at first performance. Suzy never again saw a stage she didn't want to be on – preferably in the center.

As a successful entrepreneur, she founded Suzy Prudden Studios – the first, largest and most successful toddler exercise school in New York City, a business that took her to 13 books, twenty national tours, The Today Show, Good Morning America and Ophra, along with hundreds of magazines and newspapers. She next started coaching her business hypnosis clients in how to grow their companies. On the way, she and her sister Joan Meijer-Hirschland wrote "The Itty Bitty® Weight Loss Book" and discovered a unique blend of publishing and business opportunity.

Together they formed the Itty Bitty Publishing Community which publishes Your Amazing Itty Bitty® Books – 15 Simple Informative Steps by Experts in Fields of All Kinds and matches them with opportunities for marketing that helps their writers grow their businesses as well as sell their books. At the same time she is developing her very successful workshop "Money Mind Mastery" – soon to be an Itty Bitty® Book.

JOAN MEIJER-HIRSCHLAND has been co-author for Suzy Prudden's last five books. They have discovered that the only way they can work effectively together is on a phone and more recently Skype. Working in the same room is hopelessly distracting. Several years ago, at the age of 70, Meijer discovered that she could write erotic short stories – Audiences sit up in their chairs and lean forward when she rolls onto a stage in her wheel chair and informs them she writes erotica under the a pen name – Joan Russell.

She also writes medical thrillers under the pen name John Russell, alternative histories and non-fiction under Joan Meijer and books about writing and Itty Bitty® Books under Joan Meijer-Hirschland.

www.ittybittypublishing.com

If You Liked This Book You Might Also Enjoy

- **Your Amazing Itty Bitty® Food & Exercise** Log – Suzy Prudden and Joan Meijer-Hirschland (Only available in paperback.)

- **Your Amazing Itty Bitty® Heal Your Body Book –** Patricia Pinto Garza

- **Your Amazing Itty Bitty® Marijuana Manual** – Kat Bohnsack

And Many More Itty Bitty® Books Available Online and in Paperback.